In this wonderful book, herbalist Kami McBride introduces the reader to a unique way of looking at menstruation as a 'shape shifting tool' that allows us to rethink and reshape our personal worlds. My favorite part of the book is Kami's suggestions for how to celebrate menstruation, 105 ways to be exact! This would be the perfect book for a young woman just entering her moon time, for a woman who is experiencing difficulty during menstruation or for any woman wishing to feel more empowered and creative during her monthly cycle.

– ROSEMARY GLADSTAR

Author of *Herbal Healing for Women and the Family Herbal*

Kami McBride offers us not only her extensive herbal knowledge but also her deep honoring of the feminine. 105 Ways to Celebrate Menstruation *contains wisdom, warm and earth based experience for all women to embrace. I highly recommend not only women to read this but also men who want to understand the feminine.*

– CANDIS CANTIN

Author of the *Pocket Gui*[illegible]*da*

105 Ways to Celebrate Menstruation *is so beautifully written! Some people write whole books trying to say what you have said succinctly, warmly and beautifully in just the first two pages.*

– DONNA WILSHIRE
Author of *Virgin, Mother, Crone*

105 Ways to Celebrate Menstruation *presents a useful tool for monthly acknowledgement of a little recognized aspect of our femininity. For women and young girls to tap into this primal source of power is revolutionary and a vital contribution to our health as a species.*

– MARGARET BEESON, ND
Medical Director, Yellowstone Naturopathic Clinic

In 105 Ways to Celebrate Menstruation, *herbalist Kami McBride teaches us how to let our monthly cycle become our ally and guide to healing and balance in our lives. Following Kami's suggestions we learn how to nourish and care for ourselves in deeply rewarding ways!*

– PATRICIA FREELAND, MA, CMT
Author of the *Spiritual Essence of Flowers*

105 Ways to Celebrate Menstruation *is wonder-filled with concise meaningful, thought provoking and empowering ideas for women of all ages. Kami has put into words much needed advice and suggestions to help women reclaim their menstruation as a time of power and insight to be honored and celebrated. You have created a valuable piece for generations of women.*

– JANE BOTHWELL
Director of Dandelion Herb Center

105 Ways to Celebrate Menstruation

105 Ways to Celebrate Menstruation

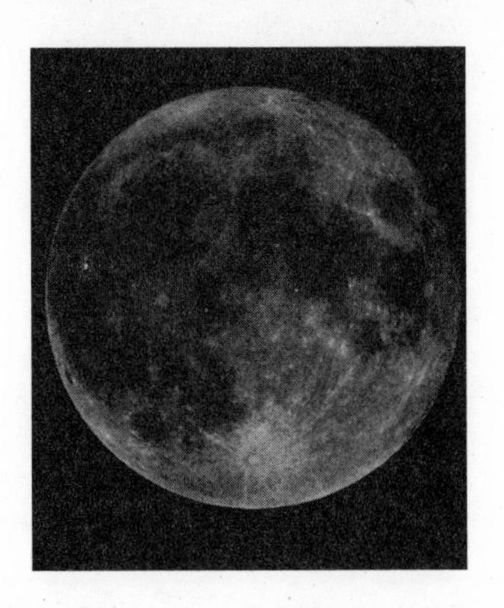

Kami McBride

105 Ways to Celebrate Menstruation

First Printing, April 2004

The purpose of this book is to educate. The information presented is in no way intended as a substitute for medical advice

Library of Congress Control Number: 2004091114

ISBN: 0-9749670-1-7

Book and cover design: Roz Abraham, Regent Press

Printed and bound in the USA

Living Awareness Publications
P.O. Box 5381
Vacaville, CA 95696
www.livingawareness.com
kami@livingawareness.com

Contents

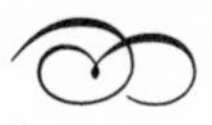

I

A New Paradigm

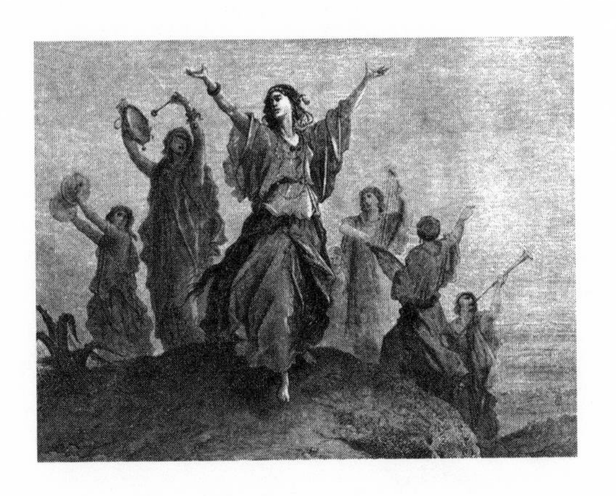

Menstruation is not usually thought of as a time of honor or celebration. It is commonly called the curse, 'that dreaded time of the month', 'a bloody mess', 'on the rag' and other derogatory names. These names are a reflection of our thoughts and feelings about menstruation. When we reject a body function as something negative, dirty or insignificant, there is an energetic and psychological separation from that part of the body. The negative thought patterns associated with menstruation are indeed part of the reason why so many women experience unique combinations of over one hundred different symptoms and ailments categorized under PMS.

We can develop a new way of thinking about menstruation. A way that creates positive thoughts and images in relation to this important body cycle. A way that allows us to truly love and accept our body just the way it is. We can learn to appreciate menstruation as something normal and healthy. When women don't feel like they have to 'do' something to hide or control this natural body function, they experience a greater sense of self esteem, well being and peace of mind.

Menstruation is a sign of good health. Without menstruation there would be no human life. The female body does its monthly cyclical dance of fluctuating hormones, releasing an egg, building tissue, thickening the uterus and then menstruating. Menstruation takes place when the body releases the uterine lining that was built up to possibly nourish a new life. Menstruation is a time of releasing and letting go in preparation to do the dance all over again.

The current primary practice in relation to menstruation is to plow through it as if nothing different is happening. The changing rhythm of our body cycle is not reflected anywhere in the calendar or work schedule. U.S. statistics show that more than fifty percent of American women are sleep deprived and we have epidemic rates of chronic fatigue and exhaustion related diseases. Menstruation is a built in cycle that provides us with the opportunity to restore and rejuvenate each month. It is a time during which the female body releases, regenerates and heals. Menstruation is a natural part of our cycle that can take us into the regenerative and contemplative aspects of the feminine. It can be helpful for a woman if she takes some personal down time to allow this process to happen in the healthiest way possible.

Many women are not consciously aware that menstruation is a resource for personal growth, balance and healing. In a culture obsessed with output and productivity, one of the gifts of the feminine is the ability to stop doing and just be. Menstruation has an inward and downward movement in the body. Part of accessing the deep wisdom of the feminine involves moving from the yang experience of outward expression and achieviment to the yin experience of going inside and listening to the deep recesses of the soul. The menstrual cycle teaches us about harmony between yin and yang, dark and light, activity and rest.

Menstruation is a time when women are more sensitive. During menstruation the uterus opens and releases. With this opening in our pelvis we become more perceptive, somewhat like the opening and increased sensitivity that occurs during pregnancy. These states of expansion that are inherent to the female cycles are one reason why women can tend to have a greater sensory awareness than men. During menstruation we are more intuitive and our psychic and sensory perceptions are heightened. Our 'over' sensitivity has been demonized when it is actually a wonderful gift.

Our culture is in great need of the wisdom that comes

through a woman's body when she drops into the deep meditative state that menstruation can invoke. It is a profoundly spiritual place from which information on how to live life can well up from within. It is not a logical place, but a place known as the feminine, a place where a woman can receive insights and inspiration.

When we listen to the wisdom that can arise from paying attention to our intuition and our bodies cyclical needs, we are guided to live our lives differently. Menstruation can lead us back to our innate body wisdom. We can reclaim the knowledge of how to truly nourish and care for ourselves during a very important aspect of being female. Imagine a world where rejuvenation, healing and spiritual connection are the experiences associated with menstruation. As we learn to deeply understand our physiology, and as we unlock the secrets of the spiritual qualities of menstruation, we will look forward to and embrace 'that time of the month'.

Instead of plugging up with tampons and drugging up with anti-inflammatories, take a little time to honor the flow of your menstrual blood. You will find that many of the problems surrounding menstruation are your body letting you know that you need to trust your irritation and fatigue and spend some time resting and allowing the body to release.

The following 105 ways to celebrate menstruation are simple suggestions that can help bring a woman back to the awareness of her cyclic nature. When a woman begins to use the rhythmic cycles of her own body to shape her world, she finds a renewed ability to maintain a healthier balance between all aspects of her life. When a woman appreciates and honors her body cycles she can awaken to a new level of the healing power of her female nature. Female energy is creative and spreading. What a woman heals within herself permeates her life and affects others around her.

As women, so much of our cyclical change goes without notice and un-celebrated. Our first menstruation, a major life transition, passes with little comment. Each month we embody the wheel of life through our menstrual cycle and for the majority of women it is considered an inconvenience at best. Menopause arrives as an event that many women just hope they survive without being too sweaty or crazy. Each of these cycles hold keys to unlocking the full potential of a woman's inner resources. It is difficult to perceive the gifts of the menstrual cycle when we basically wish it would just go away. To begin to understand the treasure held within our cycles, we first have to change our mind about how we feel about them.

Finding simple ways to acknowledge and celebrate the flow within your womb each month is a step toward honoring and loving your natural body cycles. When you love and care for your body, you experience your cycles from a more empowered context. Your monthly cycle becomes your ally, a guide to healing and balance.

As a woman you embody the seasons and cycles of the moon, the ebb and flow of the tides and the mystery of change. Enjoy these suggestions to help you experience a sense of reverence and respect for the miraculous cycles that flow through you.

II
Celebrate Your Menstruation!

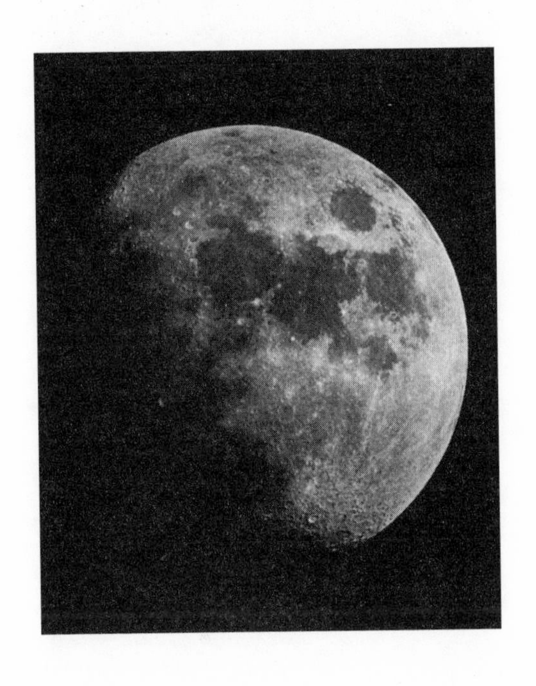

Preparation

• Create a peaceful place for you to menstruate. Dedicate a room for menstruating or when you begin bleeding, change your bed into your menstrual sanctuary with fabric and candles

• Make a menstrual altar that you set up specifically during menstruation. Have certain objects that you place on your altar during menstruation. Use your altar to support the meditative and spiritual qualities of this time

• Buy red flannel sheets for your bed

• Make a round red velvet pad that you put on your chair during menstruation

• Make a red silk herbal dream pillow to use just for

your menstrual time

• Make a beaded belt that you wear around your belly when you menstruate

• Give your bleeding vagina a special name: rose garden, dragens temple, flood gate, red door, pomegranate garden, red cave, sacred jewel, ruby lips, blossoming lotus....

• Create a special tea blend that you drink during menstruation

• Make an herbal tincture to help ease cramps

• Buy a piece of jewelry that you wear only during menstruation

• Put shells on your altar that remind you of your body's association with the moon and the ocean tides

• Read an inspirational book on women

• Buy or make a special container to keep all of your menstrual paraphernalia in, such as your cloth pads, chosen jewelry, altar objects, belly belts and any items of adornment that you use during menstruation

• Purchase a beautiful drinking glass and dinner plate that you eat and drink from only during menstruation

- Sew a soft red pouch to keep your menstrual pads in

- Track your menstruation with a calendar so you can plan a day off in advance

- Collect pictures and images of things that have been associated with menstruation: caves, volcanoes, red flowers, dragons, bowls, snakes, the ocean, the moon, cauldrons, pommegranites and fruit trees

- Make a menstrual journal by covering a notebook with fabric or pasting pictures on it that you like. Use it to record your menstrual intuitions, inspirations and dreams

- Stock your refrigerator with good food before you begin menstruating. This allows you to enjoy noursishing yourself without having to go shopping during the peak of your moontime

- Bring your emotional life into integrity before you begin bleeding. Take time to complete anything that has been building up this month. Is there something that you need to say to someone but have not done so? Try to clear your plate of recent emotional events so you can fully be with the insights of your menstrual time

- Think about your first moontime and make an offering of gratitude to your body for all your years of menstruating

• Create a Women's Wisdom circle where you meet with friends and share your experiences in relation to menstruation and all aspects of the female cycles

• Create a moon lodge. A place where bleeding women can come together and relax, support each other, sing, do herbal pampering, share stories and be together during menstruation

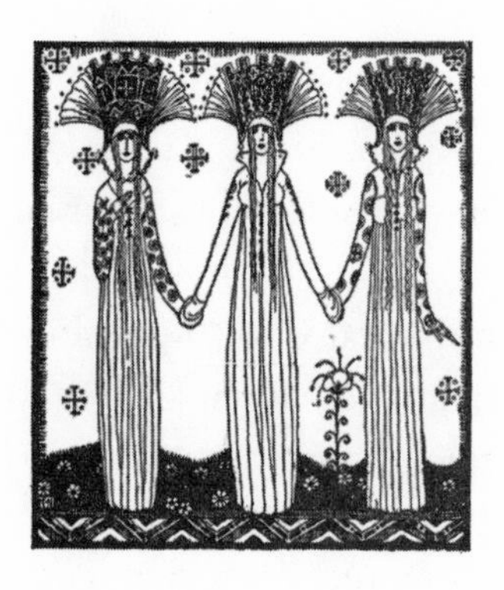

Giving to Yourself

• Give your menstrual cycle a name that invokes positive healing thoughts and images: My moon, moontime, womb time, my time, my flow, my cycle, my blood time, sacred cycle, moon cycle, sacred moon cycle, blood cycle, dragon time, red dragon, red river, red moon, red tide, high tide, ...

• Menstruation is a time of release and rejuvenation. At the beginning of each monthly blood cycle, set your intention to use the magic of your menstruation to bring healing to something in your life

• Wear red lipstick

• Paint your nails red

• Henna your hair

• Give yourself a henna tattoo

• Wear red underwear

• Wear soft cotton menstrual pads

• Menstruation is a time of regeneration. You can support your body's natural process by giving yourself permission to rest and relax. Take some time to do whatever puts you into a deeply relaxed state; gentle yoga poses, resting by the fire, massage, imagery, chanting, visualization, meditation or deep breathing. Develop relaxation tools during your non-menstrual time so that when you bleed you can easily take yourself into a very relaxed state

• Make a special meal of your favorite food

•Ask someone you love to prepare a meal of your favorite food for you

• Have a glass of red wine

• Have a glass of red juice (grape, pomegranate, cherry, cranberry, carrot, beet..)

• Eat red foods (steamed beets, beet soup, apples, pomegranates, red onion, red bell peppers, squash, cranberries, cherries, currants, raspberries, strawberries)

• Light red candles

• Sit in your menstrual space and think about what has taken place in your life between now and the last time you bled. Review the previous month and acknowledge your life experiences during this past moon cycle. Sometimes we are too busy during the month to assimilate various experiences. Use the cleansing power of your bleeding time to integrate anything that has been incomplete for you

•Take time to write in your journal. Make a list of the things that were nourishing and made you happy in the past month. Make a list of the things that have been depleting and draining to you in the past month

• Lay in bed all afternoon just sleeping and dreaming

• Squat and bleed directly onto the earth

• Wear a red beaded necklace

• Wear rubies, garnets or moonstone

• Wash your menstrual cloth pads in a small bucket or bowl. Water your house plants with the water you washed your pads in

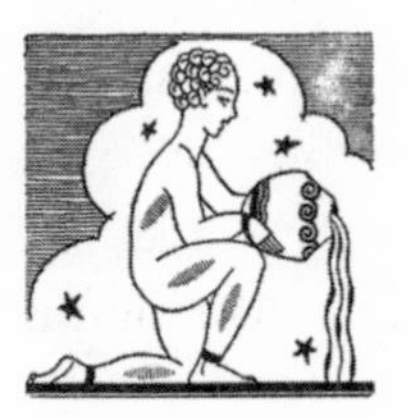

• Wash your menstrual cloth pads in a small bucket or bowl. Pour the water on your garden beds or the compost pile

• Menstruation is a time of healing and a sign of good health. Create a special blessing or prayer of gratitude that you say to yourself when you begin bleeding each month

• Put a red blanket on your bed

• Wear red earrings

• Wear a red bindi on your forehead

• Anoint your charkas with aromatherapy oils

• Get together with another bleeding woman and give each other pedicures

• Rub olive oil, sesame oil or St. John's wort oil on your low back and belly

• Find out what zodiac sign the moon is in while you are bleeding and look up the properties of that sign

• Create a quiet space and allow yourself to breathe and relax for a while. Then let yourself write unconditionally and unedited for ten minutes. Write down what your womb has to say to you. Without thinking about what you are writing, just imagine that your womb is telling you what it needs and wants. Let your womb tell you what it has to say to you about anything in your life

• If you feel irritable or angry, write down all of the things that are bothering you

• Give yourself at least two full hours of solitude

• Let the people around you know that you are menstruating

• Purchase or make an aromatic herbal oil. Rub it all over your body every day that you are bleeding. While you are massaging your body, tell it that you love it and thank your body for all that it does for you

• Eat foods and dried fruits that are traditionally associated with a woman's fertility, nurturing and ability to bear fruit: red apples, red rose petals, dates, honey, cream, pomegranates, figs, coconut and dried pears

• Take a bath with lavender and rose petals

• Go outside at night and notice what phase the moon is in while you are bleeding. Is it new or full, waning, waxing or hidden from view? Is it in a different phase than in the last time you bled?

• Burn some incense and say a healing prayer. Imagine the smoke from the incense carrying your menstrual prayers out into the world

• Menstrual blood is the substance that nourishes the beginning of human life. It is the sacred blood of life; no one is hurt when it is shed. As your blood flows out of you dedicate it as an offering of healing

• Turn off the phone and take a nice long nap

• Sit outside with your back next to a tree. Bleed directly onto the ground and feel the support of the tree along your spine

• Use your menstrual blood as paint. On a piece of paper, paint symbols that represent something you would like to release from your life, then burn the paper

• Use your menstrual blood to paint a rock. Paint symbols representing an old habit or pattern that you would like to let go of. Throw the rock into the ocean or river or bury it in the earth

• Give yourself a chamomile footbath and massage your ankles and feet with sesame oil

• Eat a bowl of organic raspberries

• Drink a lunar infusion made with healing flowers

• Find a warm and comfortable place in nature to sit and bleed on the ground

• Menstruation is a great time to work with any divination tools that are available to you; tarot cards, MOON CARDS, the I Ching, journaling, praying, astrology or whatever you use to help you look more deeply into the nature of who you are

• Have orgasms, for some women they help relieve cramps

• Wear a red skirt

• Wear a red scarf

• Wear all red clothes

• Light a candle and say prayers of appreciation for your cycle. Thank your body for connecting you to the rhythm of life. Thank it for all of your cycles, for your creative female energy and for the possible opportunity to bear a child. Thank your cycle for the gift of heightened sensitivity. Let yourself be in a space of gratitude and say thank you for whatever comes to mind about who you are

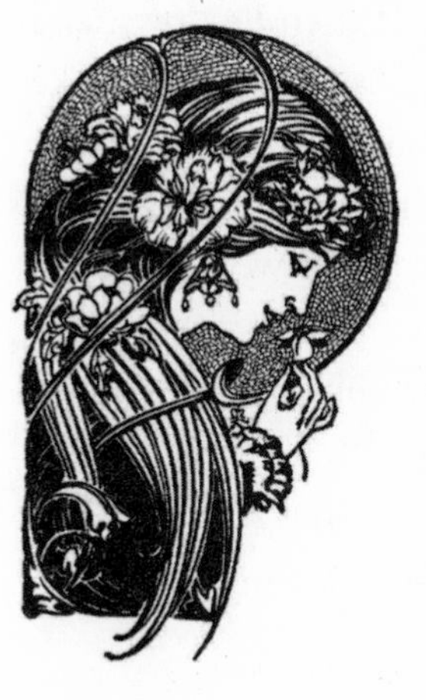

• Stay warm. Keep your feet and ankles warm

• Sit in front of your altar. Drum, rattle, chant, breathe or use whatever techniques you like that calm your mind and help you listen to your inner voice. Ask your inner voce if there is anything that you need to be aware of that you may not have been paying attention to

• Write down your dreams

•Remove yourself from all external stimulus. Find the deepest stillnes within you

• Curl up with a blanket and a cup of tea by the fire

• Do a warm herbal oil treatment on your hair

• Eat a piece of chocolate

• Find a nice smooth round rock about the size of two fists. Let it warm up in the sun and then lie down and place the rock on your belly over your womb. Make sure the rock is warm. With the rock on your belly, close your eyes and breathe deeply. Let the warmth and weight of the rock bring your attention to your womb. Notice how you feel in this part of your body. Experiment with different rocks until you find a womb rock that is the size and weight that feels best to you. Using a rock in this way is very soothing and grounding and can help you to bring your awareness deep into your womb

- Use some of your bleeding time to just be, without having to do anything

- Use colored pencils or pastels to draw any images that come in your dreams while you are bleeding

- Honor your menstrually induced heightened awareness and sensory perception. Surround yourself with pleasing colors and scents

- Turn off the television, bright lights and computer. Use soft lighting and candlelight

- Daydream

Emergence

As you reach the end of your cycle and begin to ascend from the depth and intensity of menstruation, here are some ways to celebrate and mark this transition from one part of your cycle to the next.

• Make some moon water and let the rays of the moon fill your body as you drink it

• Lie naked in the moonlight and allow the moon rays to shine between your legs

• Sing a song to the moon

• Schedule an appointment for a massage or other healing therapy at the end of your moontime

- Splash your body with rose water

- Do something that brings you joy and that you love to do

- Look at inspirational images of women and goddesses

- Have someone comb or braid your hair

- Menstruation is the state in which we cultivate our sensitivity. Write several paragraphs on how your sensitivity is beneficial to you in your life

- Make an herbal body powder and powder your entire body after you bathe. As you touch each part of your body, adore yourself, love yourself and hold the intention that you are sending messages of love and appreciation to every cell

- Lie in your bed, cozy and warm or if it is a summer night, go outside and lie in the moonlight. Close your eyes and imagine the luminescent light of the moon entering your body through the top of your head. As you breathe deeply, allow the healing energy of the moon to flow down from your head into your neck and through your body, moving all the way down into your legs and out the bottom of your feet. Let the energy of the moon wash through your body for as long as you like. Relax, rest and soak up the ancient wisdom of grandmother moon

• Create a pleasing herbal blend to bathe in at the end of your cycle. Do this to signify your re-emergence into the world

• Light a candle. Ask yourself, "What is my image of what is sacred, valuable, reverent and holy about being a woman?"

• Menstruation is a time of accessing a deeper knowing about who we are. Ask yourself, "What pearl of wisdom am I re-emerging with?"

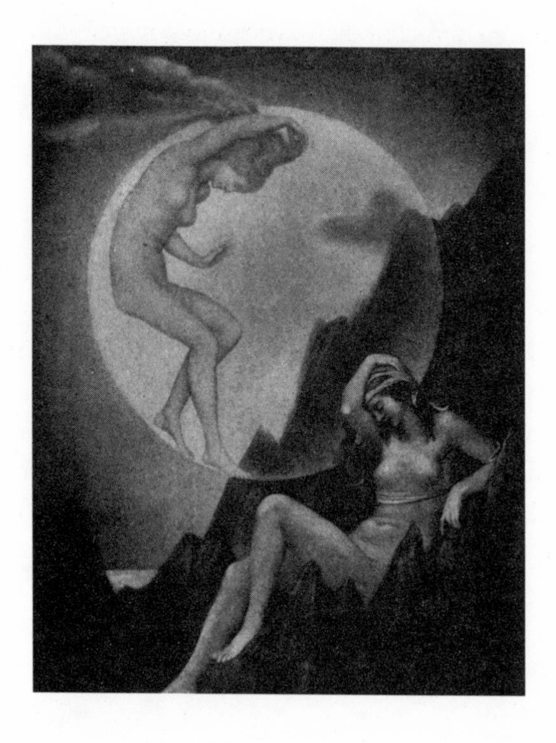

Ideas for Celebrating Menstruation:

III

Celebrating with the Gifts of the Earth

Tea

Put herbal combinations into water in a stainless steel or enamel pot. With the lid on the pot, bring the herb(s) to a boil and then turn off the heat and let the herbs continue to steep for two hours. Re-heat the tea when you are ready to use it.

High Tide Tea
3 cups water
1 tablespoon dandelion leaf
1 tablespoon oatstraw
1 tablespoon chamomile
1 teaspoon raspberry leaf
1 teaspoon rose petals
1 teaspoon ginger root

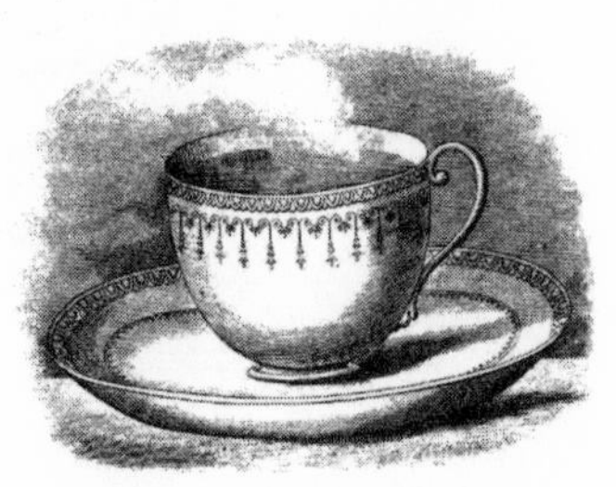

Calming the Moon Tea

3 cups water

1 tablespoon chamomile

1 tablespoon passionflower

1 tablespoon lemonbalm

New Moon Tea

2 cups water

1 tablespoon rose petals

1 tablespoon hibiscus

1/8 teaspoon cinnamon

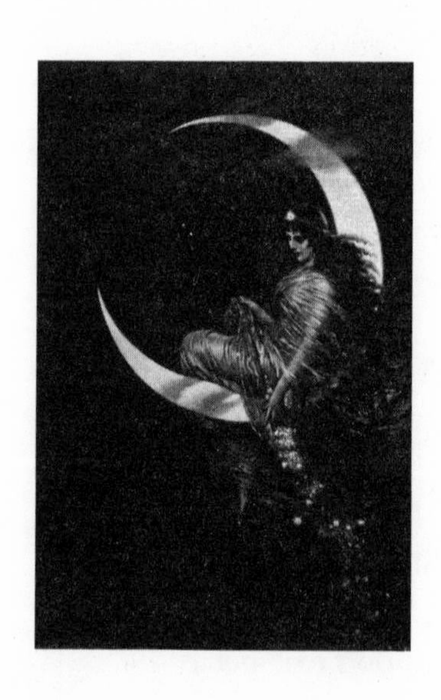

Lunar Tea

Put four cups of water and four tablespoons of dried herbs or eight tablespoons of fresh herbs into a glass quart mason jar and put the lid on. Let the jar sit out under the moonlight over night. In the morning, strain out the herbs and drink the infusion or pour it into your bath. The shelf life of this infusion is two to three days and it can be stored in the refrigerator.

Healing Lunar Flower Tea
4 cups water
1 tablespoon lavender flowers
1 tablespoon violet flowers
1 tablespoon borage flowers
1 tablespoon elder flower

Full Moon Tea
4 cups water
1 tablespoon mugwort leaf/flower
1 tablespoon rose petals
1 tablespoon elder flowers
1 teaspoon rosemary
1 teaspoon chamomile

Moonwater

Pour some fresh clean filtered or unchlorinated water into a large glass bowl. Put it outside in a place where the moon can shine into the water overnight. Drink or bathe with the water the next day.

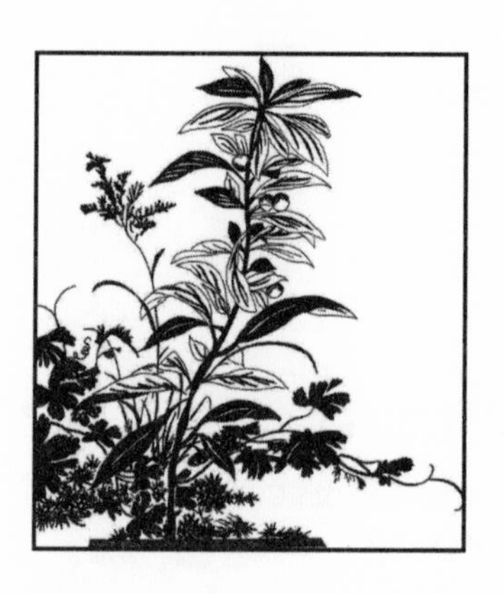

Herbal Baths

Make four gallons of tea in a large canning pot. Heat the tea and pour it directly into the bathtub. If you don't want a big mess to clean up, strain the herbs from the tea before pouring it into the bathtub. Then wrap the herbs into a pouch using a piece of cotton cloth and a string or rubber band tied around it. Put the tea and the pouch of herbs into the bathwater.

The Menstrual Bath

4 gallons water
1/2 cup lavender leaf/flower
1/2 cup rose petals
1/2 cup chamomile
1/4 cup anise hyssop leaf/flower
1 cup whole oats

Moon Bath

4 gallons water
1 cup mugwort flowers
1 cup lemon balm leaf

Re-emergence Bath

4 gallons water
1/2 cup rosemary
1/2 cup calendula
1/4 cup yarrow
1/4 cup sage

Footbaths

Make teas out of the following recipes and do not strain out the herbs. Pour the tea and herbs into a foot basin. Once the tea has cooled to a comfortable temperature, put both feet into the basin Let your feet soak for as long as you like.

Womb time Footbath

6 cups water
2 tablespoons rosemary
2 tablespoons lavender
2 tablespoons mugwort

Invigorating Footbath

6 cups water
2 tablespoons rosemary
2 tablespoons eucalyptus leaf
2 tablespoons peppermint

Sleepy Time Footbath

6 cups water
3 tablespoons chamomile
2 tablespoons hops
1 tablespoon skullcap

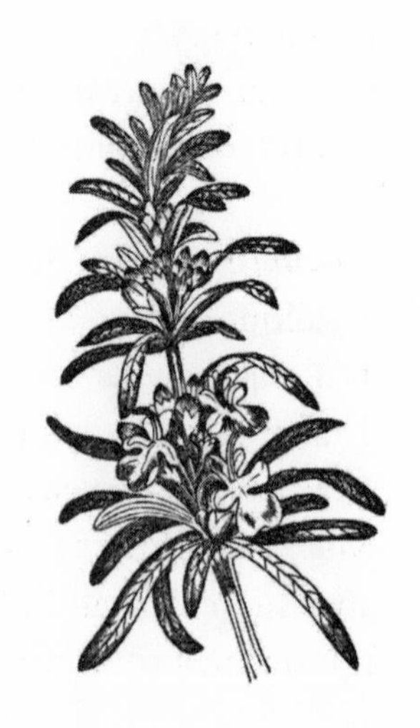

Foot Scrubs

Increasing circulation in the feet and keeping them warm helps to ease menstrual difficulties. Herbal foot scrubs are a combination of herbs mixed with other exfoliating ingredients like salt, ground nuts and powdered grains. Rub the foot scrubs onto the feet in small circular motions for five to fifteen minutes. Leave the scrub on for another five to ten minutes, more or less depending on how it feels to you.

Heating Foot Scrub

4 tablespoons rice powder
(powder rice kernals in a blender)
1 tablespoon ground sunflower seeds
2 teaspoons clove
2 teaspoons ginger
2 teaspoons coriander
1 teaspoon cinnamon

Powder each ingredient separately and then mix together. Add just enough olive oil to make a paste and rub it onto the feet.

Circulation! Foot Scrub

1/4 cup Epsom salts
1/4 cup sea salt
2 tablespoons dried powdered ginger root
5 drops juniper essential oil

Mix ingredients together and add 1/8 cup of olive oil and mix thoroughly. Massage the salts on the feet for up to fifteen minutes.

Pleasure Foot Scrub

1 cup sea salt

2 tablespoons powdered orange peel

1 tablespoon powdered lemongrass

1/8 cup lavender infused herbal oil

2 drops ylang ylang essential oil

Mix ingredients together thoroughly. Massage the salts on the feet for up to fifteen minutes.

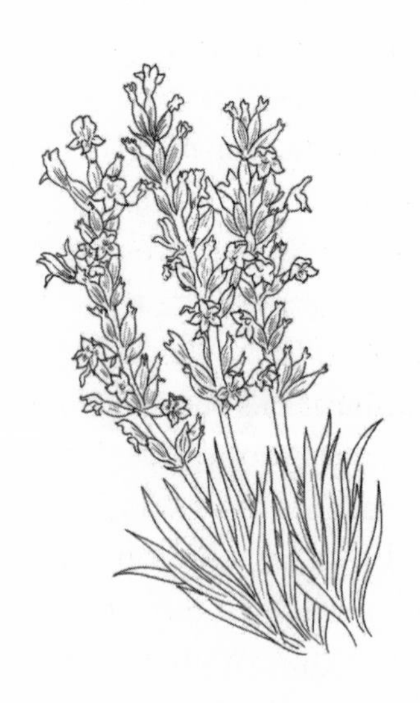

HERBAL TINCTURES

There are many ways to make herbal tinctures. The following recipe is very effective for menstrual cramps and can easily be made in your own kitchen. A cordial is simply an herbal tincture that has ingredients added such as fruit and honey to make the tincture sweet.

Moontime Cramp-Ease Cordial
4 tablespoons dried cramp bark herb
1 tablespoon hops flowers
1 tablespoon California poppy leaf/flower
1 teaspoon orange peel
1/8 teaspoon cinnamon
1/4 cup fresh or frozen organic raspberries
1/8 cup raisins
Brandy
Vodka
Honey
Chop ingredients together. Mix your alcohol so that it is equal parts brandy and 100 proof vodka, so mix half vodka and half brandy together. Cover the herbal combination with twice as much of the alcohol mixture as herbal ingredients. Let it sit for one month shaking it occasionally. Using a cotton cloth, strain the herb and fruit mixture out of the liquid. Discard the fruit and herbs. Add three tablespoons of honey or more to taste to the liquid. Take 1-2 teaspoons up to five times a day as needed. This is a very sedating and relaxing herbal remedy. Driving is not recommended.

Infused Herbal Oil

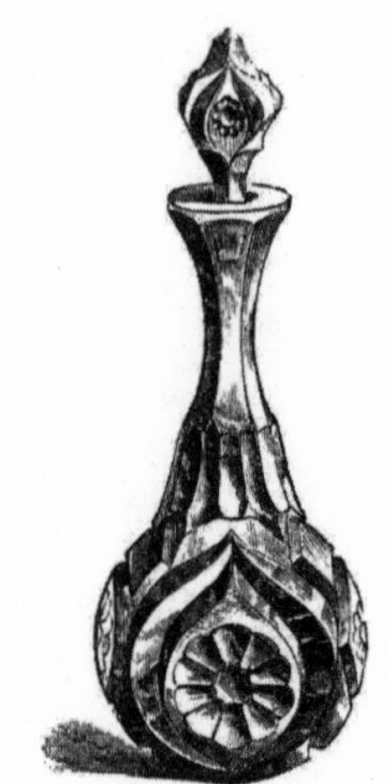

Ruby Moon Foot Oil

2 cups olive oil

1/2 cup lavender leaf/flower

1/2 cup St. John's wort leaf/flower

1/4 cup calendula flower

Mix ingredients together in the blender. Let sit for four weeks and strain the herbs from the oil.

Mugwort oil

1 cup olive oil

1/2 cup fresh or dried mugwort

Mix ingredients together in the blender and let sit for four weeks. Strain the herbs out and store in a cool dry place. This is great oil for cramps, coldness, low back tension and pain.

Sacred Cycle Anointing Oil

4 ounces of infused herbal oil of st. John's wort

2 drops myrrh essential oil

2 drops jasmine essential oil

Mix the essential oils into the St. John's wort base oil

Shimmering Moon Hair Oil

2 tablespoons infused rosemary herbal oil

2 tablespoon infused calendula herbal oil

2 tablespoons infused nettles herbal oil

1 tablespoon sesame oil

Place oils together in a double boiler on very low heat and add 1 tablespoon of shea butter. After all ingredients are melted together add 5 drops rosemary essential oil. Begin with a clean sterilized jar and finely chopped dried herbs. Loosely powder the herbs using a regular kitchen blender. Put two cups of dried herbs into a quart jar and then fill the jar to the top with olive oil. Let this sit for two to four weeks in a cabinet, shaking the mixture occasionally. Then strain the herbs from the oil.

Bleeding Woman Belly Oil

2 1/2 cups olive oil
1/2 cup castor oil
1/2 cup mugwort leaf/flower
1/2 cup St. John's wort leaf/flower
1/2 cup chamomile
1 teaspoon 100 proof vodka
Mix ingredients together in the blender and let sit for four weeks and strain the herbs from the oil.

Love Your Body Butter

1/4 cup infused herbal oil of chamomile
1/4 cup infused herbal oil of st. John's wort
1/4 cup jojoba oil
2/3 cup cocoa butter
2 tablespoons beeswax
Heat ingredients together over low heat in a double boiler. After all ingredients are in a liquid state pour them into a glass jar. As mixture cools, add 5 drops of blue chamomile essential oil.

Herbal Body Powder

Herbal body powders are very easy to make and do not contain the chemicals that many of the cosmetic powders do. One of the simple pleasures in life is powdering your body after a nice long herbal bath.

Moontime Protection Powder

1/2 cup cornstarch
1/2 cup rice flour
1/8 cup finely powdered yarrow
1/8 cup finely powdered roses
3 drops of cedar essential oil

Moondust Body Powder

1/2 cup white clay
1/4 cup cornstarch
1/8 cup finely powdered mugwort
1/8 cup finely powdered lavender
1/8 cup finely powdered sage

Herbal Pillows

Make a pillow with soft red fabric that is about 9 inches by 4 inches in size and fill with dried herbs

Red Tide Dream Pillow

2 tablespoons hops

2 tablespoons rose petals

1 tablespoon lavender flowers

1 tablespoon mugwort

Sleepy Time Herb Pillow

2 tablespoons chamomile

2 tablespoons lavender

2 tablespoons lemon balm

Red Foods

Red Moon Juice

Put into a juicer

4 carrots

1 beet

1 apple

Small slice of ginger

Red Raspberry Smoothie

1 cup organic frozen or fresh raspberries

1/2 cup yogurt

1 cup hibiscus tea

One teaspoon powdered rose hips

One teaspoon powdered hawthorne berries

Pinch of cinnamon

Pinch of cardamom

Beet Red Soup

4 chopped beets

4 stocks of celery

3 carrots

1 leek

1 small to medium sized acorn squash with the skin and seeds removed and cut into squares

One large onion

4 cloves garlic

2 tablespoons powdered thyme

2 tablespoons powdered rosemary

2 tablespoons fresh parsley

2 tablespoons fresh dandelion leaf
Dash of salt and pepper
1 bay leaf
1 burdock root
4 pieces of astragalus

In a large pot, sauté onions, garlic, thyme in a little olive oil and water for 5 minutes. Add 3 quarts of water and put in celery, leek, carrots, acorn squash, beets, bay leaf, rosemary, burdock root, salt, pepper and astragalus. Simmer until vegetables are at the desired consistency. Take 4 cups of the soup and blend it in a blender and add it back to the stock. Garnish with freshly chopped parsley and dandelion leaf.

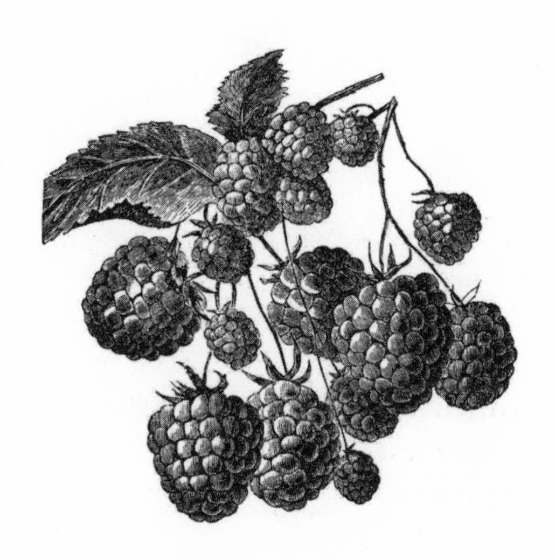

Notes:

Resources

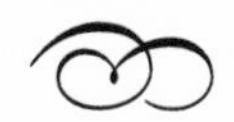

HERBS

Look for local resources in your area such as herb shops and health food stores.

Mail Order Herbs

Mountain Rose Herbs	800-879-3337
Dry Creek Herb Farm	530-888-0889
Wild Weeds	800-553-9453

Herbal Oils

Oak Grove Herbals 707-446-1290
    Healing breast oils, and St. John's wort oil
Alchemy Botanicals 541-488-4118

Moon Cards

Inspirational deck of 63 cards to support menstruation
707-446-1290
www.livingawareness.com

Cloth Menstrual Pads

Glad Rags	503-282-0436
Goddess Moons	877-551-1326
	www.goddessmoons.com
Reddy's Cloth Pads	415-485-3824
	www.reddyspads.com

About the Author

Kami McBride is a practicing herbalist in Vacaville, CA, and has taught herbal medicine and women's health since 1988. Kami has studied plants for almost 20 years and her popular course, Cultivating the Herbal Medicine Woman Within is an experiential earth awareness and herbal studies program for women. Kami's courses provide a sanctuary for women to transform their relationship with their body and remember their heritage as healers and herbalists. She is also the creator of MOON CARDS, inspirational cards to honor menstruation.

Kami can be reached at www.livingawareness.com

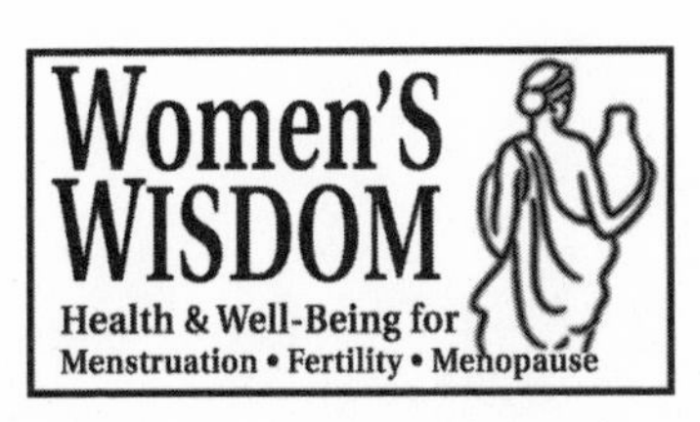

Join Kami McBride in this transformational workshop that empowers women to take charge of thier body and make informed choices about their changing cycles. Menstruation, ovulation and menopause are a continuum of experience. A healthy menarche (first menstruation) and menstrual well-being prepare you for a vital menopause and post menopause experience. Women's Wisdom is gained through a woman's intimate relationship and understanding of her body. This knowledge was once passed from woman to woman and is virtually absent in today's society. Now each phase of a woman's cycle is usually learned in a crash course fashion and there is really no place that a woman truly learns about the complexities of her female nature and body cycles.

- Turn menstruation into an experience of celebration, love and renewal for your body
- Experience menopause as a powerful and healing time in your life
- Learn the skills to prepare young women for a healthy first menstruation

Please call for upcoming
Women's Wisdom workshop dates
707-446-1290